Herbal Medicine Insomnia:

The 10 Best Solutions to Solve Insomnia Naturally

recorded copy and is only allowed with an expressed written consent from the Publisher. All additional rights reserved.

The information in the following pages is broadly considered to be truthful and accurate account of facts, and as such any inattention, use or misuse of the information in question by the reader will render any resulting actions solely under their purview. There are no scenarios in which the publisher or the original author of this work can be in any fashion deemed liable for any hardship or damages that may befall them after undertaking information described herein.

Additionally, the information in the following pages is intended only for informational purposes and should thus be thought of as universal. As befitting its nature, it is presented without assurance regarding its prolonged validity or interim quality. Trademarks that are mentioned are done without written consent and can in no way be considered an endorsement from the trademark holder.

Table of Contents

Introduction

Congratulations on downloading *Herbal Medicine Insomnia: The 10 Best Solutions to Solve Insomnia Naturally* and thank you for doing so.

The following chapters will discuss why insomnia happens in the first place and what are the best natural solutions that there are to combat against it and keep it away for good. Inside this book you will find not only what are the 10 best natural herbs used to overcome insomnia, but several other handy tips as well that you can use for the rest of your life. Herbal teas that help to bring on a good night's sleep will be discussed, as well as why it is a good idea to have certain plant life hanging in the room that you sleep in. You will also get to learn exactly what the circadian clock is and how you can begin to get yours in tune with Mother Nature and her celestial children that are the sun and moon.

The title of the book may say *10 Best solutions*, but more than only 10 tips will be found within its pages. You will learn about the 10 best herbs to use to defeat insomnia, but plenty of other information that can be used in conjunction with those 10 herbs will be given to you.

There are plenty of books on this subject on the market, thanks again for choosing this one! Every effort was made to ensure it is full of as much useful information as possible, please enjoy!

Chapter 1:

Why Can't You Sleep?

Roughly about 60 million people in the United States suffer from the sleep malady known as insomnia. That is only accounting for one country. Across the entire world insomnia is estimated to disrupt the sleep of about a third of the entire populace. If you were wondering if you were the only one who wasn't capable of getting a solid night's rest, you can be sure that you are not alone.

Insomnia may very well be the oldest of all human conflictions. Since sleeping is as old as mankind, tracing the origins of insomnia back to the original source is an impossible mystery to unravel. Even more, insomnia will most likely never be an affliction that just ups and goes away.

As long as there is a human race that needs sleep, there will be insomnia to disrupt it.

Sleep and nature have always shared a very special one of a kind of relationship between each other. The intricate delicacy of this relationship can even be said to be reflective of the process known as evolution and involution. This may sound like a stretch, but the purpose of this book is not just to simply teach you about using different herbs for the sole sake of defeating the cowardly and multifarious, hellish thief of sleep that has been called insomnia. It is much more than that. The purpose of this book is to pull you out of the mundane doldrums that is our modern day rat race of a society and its opulent amount of distractions. The point of this book may be focused on how to use herbs to get better sleep, but that is (like so many things in life) only a thinly veiled simulacrum that is hiding the real truth. The real purpose of this book is to get you back in touch with the glory and splendor that has given birth to every man, woman, child, beast, plant, mineral, grain, atom, and subatomic particle.

The real purpose of this book is to reintroduce you to Mother Nature, for without her constant effort and guidance you would not be here. There would be no planet earth or any other celestial body floating out there in the recess of stellar space. There would be no solar system. There would be no time, space, or time-space. This book would not exist without Mother Nature. No author would have ever constructed a thought to put down in writing. No language would have ever developed. No society would have ever grown out of the mud and waters, later to tower onwards reaching ever closer to the rim of the atmosphere that surrounds our planet. There would be no evolution. There would be no concept of spirit. There would be no sun to wake up to, and no moon to sleep under.

You may think that such an intro is misleading or exaggerated. Well, I would tell you to sleep on it, but we are not there yet. I'm sure that after you put all the information in this book to practical use and you do get some solid sleep, then these words will return to you later and revelation will come. That time has not come yet, though, first you need to learn why insomnia happens in the first place and figure out where something may have gone wrong with your circadian clock. If you are not sure how insomnia may have snuck up on you or are wondering what in the blazes a circadian clock is, then get ready to learn a whole lot more than just that.

Take Sleep Seriously

The average person will, and is supposed to, spend almost have of their lifetime asleep. Reading that may sound factious but if you think about it you will realize it's not. We are up during the daylight hours going to work, being with friends and family, enjoying our hobbies and doing everything that we have to get done before the sun dips away. During those hours we are expending energy and (for many of us) letting our minds run at a frantic pace just to keep up with the current tides. The old axiom of *"There just aren't enough hours in the day."*, is a phrase that many learn to eventually accept as a cold and hard truth. However, there is an ancient trick to reconciling this age-old problem. It is the oldest trick in every book and has been extolled time and time again. The best way to manage your time better during the day, and harness your energy to its fullest potential, is to get a solid 6-8 hours of sleep the night before.

It may be a small tip that you are already aware of, but for the sake of being as comprehensive as possible, you should be getting at least six hours of sleep every night. That is a lowball number, as 8 hours is what just about every medical professional recommends. Even if your schedule doesn't seem to allow it you must make time to receive the proper amount of sleep. If you like to watch television late at night, gallivant around town, or find any other reasons to avoid getting the proper amount of sleep you will have to start altering that before doing anything else. The more sleep you get in the evening, the more hours you have to do what you want the following day. As difficult as this may be to hear, this also applies to business and social engagements. It may seem like the responsible decision is to skip a few hours of sleep, so you can fit more time in to get work done- but it's not. The true responsible decision is to get more and better sleep, so you can work to your fullest ability the following day. This applies to social engagements as well. You may not want to miss out on all the fun or opportunities that seem to come with networking and fraternizing, but if you do not receive the proper amount of sleep then you just won't be your sharpest and most lucid when going to those social engagements. It's a tradeoff that may not seem fair but getting the right amount of sleep is truly the most responsible decision you can make for yourself and those around you.

Sleeping is the most natural way for the body to repair itself. The benefits of getting good sleep cannot be argued. There is a very good reason why doctors often recommend getting plenty of bed rest when someone has a cold or is recovering from an operation. The cells of our bodies repair themselves when we lay down to sleep. A cut on the flesh will not quickly heal unless the body reverts into the "sleep state". When in sleep state, our muscles know it is time to relax and not expend energy, instead harnessing it so it can be utilized the next day. While we are recollecting our energy, maintenance is being performed on those muscles, and our organs as well. The human immune system can become confused when it does not get enough sleep, and when it becomes confused it may not do the work of repairing our bodies the best it should. This is why sleep is something that needs to be taken seriously.

Sleep is not just a necessity for our bodies and cells to repair themselves but is just as important for the mind. We don't just expend physical energy while running around during the day, but mental energy as well. A plethora of thoughts and conflictions, tough decisions and judgment calls, can swell up and leave a festering hive of confusion and stress in our minds. During sleep our minds also have a chance to settle down, turnoff so to speak, and calm down the volatile ocean of scattered thoughts. This is where the phrase, *"Let me sleep on that."*, originates from. It is far easier to make a hard decision after getting a good night's sleep, and also easier to work out the cacophony of stress that has built up during the day.

The human subconscious gets to shine during sleep. Ask any psychologist and they will tell you that the subconscious is not something we can directly interact with on any practical or rationale level. It needs to sort things out for itself without the self-consciousness getting in its way. The only chance it gets to do that and work on its own is while we sleep. The pile of ideas, fears, hopes, and everything else that we encountered and thought of during a normal day would only grow higher and more unstable if not for the subconscious settling things in order while in sleep. This may seem like common knowledge but, before going any further in this book, ask yourself a very important question…

"Do I take sleep seriously enough?"

The reason this question is so important is because, when asking it with astute clarity, you are projecting a direct message to your body, and mind. Since sleeping is not just physical but also mental, creating the right frame of mind before diving into the tips and herbs used to defeat insomnia is paramount. This idea of creating the proper mindset for sleep will be more valuable to some than for others. If your insomnia has been caused due to a purely physical condition, then many of the herbs and tips in this book may be enough to help you. If, however, your insomnia is due to a mental condition then creating the right frame of mind, one that moves you away from insomnia, will be just as important if not more than any advice you will receive here or anywhere else. Thankfully, the herbs you will learn about in this book are all conducive to not just relaxing your tensions and nerves, but also to inducing the proper frame of mind needed to get a good night's rest.

Why Does Insomnia Happen?

One of the biggest problems with trying to combat insomnia is figuring out why you can't fall or stay asleep in the first place. When most people first experience insomnia they don't even realize that they have a problem. They will usually think that it was just one bad day, spiraling into one bad night of (or lack of) sleep and write it off. Then it happens again, and again, until they realize that they have fallen into a very unwanted pattern. It's sad to say, but most people take sleep for granted until they have been bitten by the bug of insomnia. Due to this combination of taking sleep for granted and not noticing that insomnia has happened before it has become a pattern, a large number of people don't ever learn why they became insomniacs in the first place.

One of the most major reasons that insomnia begins is due to medical conditions. If you are positive that your insomnia is because of a medical condition, consult your doctor along with following the guidance of this book. Sometimes the medical condition alone may be causing insomnia, while in other cases it may only be the symptoms of a condition that are causing it. Check the list below to see if your situation matches anything you see.

- Asthma
- Pain in the lower back
- Sinus or nasal allergies
- Arthritis
- Chronic pain (of any sort)
- Gastrointestinal issues (such as acid reflux)
- Sleep Apnea

Those are only a few of the more common medical conditions that can cause insomnia. Along with those, there can also be neurological conditions (like *Parkinson's Disease or restless leg syndrome)* or a large number of different conflictions that may prevent the brains neurotransmitters from operating correctly.

Aside from medical conditions, many choices that we make, and lifestyle decisions can prevent our brains from being able to calm down and find their sleep state.

- Too much caffeine
- Alcohol (may help to fall asleep, but not stay asleep)
- Graveyard shifts at work
- Working from home
- Diet (not just what you eat, but when)

Then there are the mental reasons for developing insomnia.

- Depression
- Tension
- Anxiety
- Overall worrying (about the past and future)

Every mental reason for people not being able to fall asleep all boil down to one point; not being able to silence the chatter and turn the brain off. Of course, it doesn't really shutdown when going to sleep but that is how you should think of it if a mental reason is the cause for your insomnia. If you are dealing with depression or any other mental condition and believe that it is linked to your insomnia then you should consult the proper professional source along with using the herbs listed in this book. Either way, if you can find a way to silence the mental noise and fall asleep, that will only help to alleviate your insomnia as well. It may be a struggle but know that it can be done. Remember that you are not alone in dealing with this problem. It is the oldest confliction to trouble mankind, and there has always been a collection of natural herbs to help you and everyone overcome these hurdles.

Nature vs Pharmacy

Over-the-counter sleeping aids are one of the most common things people reach for when trying to move out of the pattern of insomnia. Pharmaceutical sleeping aids do have their place, if they didn't work to some extent then people wouldn't spend billions of dollars on them every year. Over-the-counter sleep aids are not all they are cracked up to be though. The list of side effects for anyone of them can be staggering to read through. In the long run, a pharmaceutical sleep aid can actually serve to hurt your sleeping pattern and lock you deeper into a cycle of insomnia. This can happen because sleep aids can be addicting. When someone stops taking the sleep aid, they will notice that they can't fall back asleep, and then start taking the sleep aid again. All-natural herbs on the other hand, when used correctly, are safe from these problems. Herbs are a substance directly handed down to us from Mother Nature herself. She has placed down these gifts for us so that we can, while navigating the courses of our daily lives, get the proper rest we all need. Much in the same way that many people take sleep for granted, the herbs that have always been with us tend to be neglected as well. Or, and possibly more common, they have not so much been neglected as they have just been unknown. When you know what herbs to use, you won't need to reach for the sleeping pills anymore.

Chapter 2:

Setting the Circadian Clock

Living organisms have a built-in internal clock that we are all born with. It is called the circadian clock. This birth given time piece helps our bodies to distinguish between the external and internal functions of our physiology based around the 24 hours of the day. There was a time, long ago before we were surrounded by light bulbs and electrical devices, where the circadian clocks of most people were left to settle themselves out without any active intervention on anyone's part. Then as technology advanced, we have slowly introduced a steady string of unnatural frequencies into our bodies and threw off the stability and integrity of our circadian clocks. Computer screens, tablets, even the cell phones most of us carry around all day can send

subtle and sinuous currents into our bodies and confuse our internal functions to the point where our circadian clocks don't really know what time it is anymore. These items, the computers and cell phones, should not be thought of as anything negative, for they do add helpful conveniences into our daily lives, but they do come with a tradeoff of misaligning our circadian clocks.

Not everything regarding the circadian clock has to do with modern technology though. Everyone is different, and the genes we are born with also have a factor in determining how well our circadian clocks operate. Somewhere up to 1 different genes have an effect in how our circadian clocks function from person to person. Some people are morning people while others will feel more clarity and surges of energy during the nighttime hours. Our individual circadian clocks will tell our bodies when it's time for rest or, when we should get up and expend energy.

Even though we are born with different gears inside our internal clocks, many people today don't even realize that theirs has been thrown out of loop with nature. Long hours at work, fighting against sleep to get other things done, jetlag, and a host of other factors can confuse our circadian clocks and thus, lead to insomnia. Even something as simple as having a small bite to eat in the later hours of the evening can confuse our clocks. When the circadian clock begins to get confused, it will still do what it can to regulate itself and possibly make a biological miscalculation while doing so. As with many of the other reasons that can cause insomnia, the vicious loop of not being able to quiet our minds and ease our bodies when we should be asleep can begin without any of us even realizing that a problem has begun.

It can be difficult to figure out if any of this has happened to you and determine for a fact that having a confused circadian clock is contributing to your lack of sleep at night. Just so you know, if

you live in our modern age (which you obviously do) and have trouble sleeping at night, then your circadian clock is properly at least somewhat maladjusted. This is nothing to feel down about as it is just a spandrel of the age and times we live in. Almost everyone has a maladjusted circadian clock nowadays. Yet, again, our biological time piece doesn't realize that something is wrong. It's not up to the circadian clock to be completely accurate and fix itself, for that will keep on ticking and tracking time along with our organs as it sees fit. It is up to us to reset the circadian clock, after recognizing that is has been thrown out of synch with the sun and moon.

Even if you don't have an inaccurate circadian clock, you should go about making sure that it ticks along as correctly as possible. To do this, you will have to reset your circadian clock and get it back on the proper time track with Mother Nature. Quick fix fads that guarantee to solve everything for you probably won't do what they claim, except take your money. Also, any pill for the most part will not correctly set your circadian clock to its proper state either. In fact, depending on what the pill is, like a sleeping pill, they will only cause to confuse your biological time tracker even more. The exceptions to this are melatonin and magnesium- which are both natural supplements and are produced inside our bodies.

Both melatonin and magnesium can help to ease muscles and relax the mind. Melatonin is often recommended when trying to induce more sleep by the medical community. Using either one of these correctly can help to reset your circadian clock, but there are other tips that you can start practicing even before reaching for those supplements.

How to reset the circadian clock

The most fundamental way to get back in tune with nature is to be aligned with the sun and moon. This is practical and conventional wisdom. We receive all of our energy from the sun and its light. Moonlight, valuable in its own regard, is only a reflection and does not send down surges of energy into our molecular cells. We should live the course of our lives with the basic system of sunlight and moonlight engrained into our minds at all times. When it is daytime, things should be bright, and during the night, things should be dark. Both, light and darkness, are necessary for our bodies to function properly.

When waking up in the morning (or just getting out of bed if you couldn't get any sleep) the first thing you should do is surround yourself with as much light as possible. Open the blinds and let the light flood your room. Open the window while you are at it to bring in some fresh air (remember that the sun also help supply oxygen). If you can, take a step outside before getting most other things done and just take a brief moment to wrap yourself in sunlight, and feel appreciation for it. Turn the lights on all over your house, especially in the room you woke up in. If you wake up very early before the sun has fully rose, it's raining outside, or the clouds are covering the sunlight, then you are going to have to rely on artificial light even more to help get your circadian clock back in proper tune with nature. Artificial light may not be as energy inducing, and of course not as natural, as sunlight, but it is better than wallowing the morning hours away while covered in darkness. The brighter your surroundings are after waking up, the more you are telling your body and mind that it is time to use energy and become lucid. If after first getting up and everything is dark, then you are sending the exact opposite message to your circadian clock. This can be one of the major reasons why many people don't feel refreshed and ready to go after getting out of bed. They wake up, and both their bodies and minds still think that it's time to get rest and slow down instead of taking action and speed up.

This same logic applies to nighttime as well. During the night it is better to lower the lights and lessen the energy. Our society is counterintuitive to this concept, in some locations. Cities are primarily guilty of creating environments where the cycle of day and night is mixed-up. Living within a *"City that never sleeps"* is not the best place to be when trying to combat insomnia. Of course, living in a city does not mean there is no hope, but if you do then it may take a little bit longer to reset your circadian clock back to being in tune with Mother Nature. If you do live in a city or some other highly populated area with a vibrant and active nightlife, be aware that you may have to put in a bit of extra effort and have patience. Remember that sleep is to be taken seriously and some of your nighttime adventures may need to be put on pause while you are trying to reset your circadian clock.

When night comes it is best to lower the volume of light surrounding you. You don't need to drape your home in total darkness but dimming the lights will begin to tell your body that it does not need to expend as much energy. Have less lights on and if you can then only try to use a few lamps. If your lights have dim switches and lower settings, use those after the sun goes down.

During the day, have your home and environment emulate the sun. During the night, emulate the moon. By doing this you will be on the way to having your body and mind emulate our most intrinsic celestial bodies, then you will be on your way to getting your circadian clock back in the proper tune with Mother Nature.

What to Do at Night

As it gets closer to bedtime you can perform a variety of different things to wind yourself down and inform the circadian clock that the time to go to sleep is getting closer. One of the best ways to accomplish this is to take a warm bath an hour or so before trying to get some sleep. Taking a warm bath has a tendency to calm the mind and relax the body. Also, warming up the body will begin to let muscles ease tension and relax.

Turn off all electric lights when it is time to go to sleep. Computers, cell phones, televisions, tablets, video game systems, and whatever else that may produce blue or red lights should be shutdown. You may even want to take the extra step and unplug these things to stifle any electric currents that may be disrupting your sleep without you even realizing it. Don't worry, when morning comes you can turn everything back on and use all the devices you want to your hearts content.

Read a book in bed or write in a journal before going to sleep. Doing these things *in bed* is key here. Reading can help to focus the mind and slow it down while at the same time putting it to a little bit extra work of processing information. Journaling can help to organize the activities and thoughts of the day that may be preventing you from quieting the mind while trying to fall asleep. If you read or write using an electrical device, just be sure to turn it off after you have finished.

Both reading, and writing can also give you something to focus on while you transition from being awake into subconsciousness, and that leads to another tip. When trying to sleep, it is not advisable to have your thoughts scattered all over the place, as that will only keep the mind too active. When trying to sleep, either focus on a memory (like a conversation) or play out a sequence in your head. The sequence could also be a memory, or even something you saw in a movie. It's also not the worst idea to let your imagination run away a tad while trying to go to sleep. Whatever your wildest fantasies may be, go ahead and envision yourself accomplishing them.

Regular exercise can do wonders for fixing the circadian clock. Try to exercise at least 45 minutes, four days out of the week. But, don't exercise right before going to sleep as that will rev you up too much.

Meditation is an excellent thing to do before going to bed. It can help to calm the mind and center your thoughts before bed.

Try not to have any caffeine 6 hours before bedtime. Also, watch the carbs after 9 pm.

Get a routine before going to bed. Having a set routine will, after a week or two, let your circadian clock know that it is time to wind down and get some shuteye.

Chapter 3:

Sleeping with Plants

It is no secret that being close to nature can help to settle down the nerves and bring a calming energy to the mind. When trying to tune in closer to Mother Nature's frequency the best thing you can do without question is spend time outside in the sunlight and take in as much of her splendor as you can. Going on a hiking trail, a park, or simply just gardening in your own yard all have the ability to bring a Zenlike breath of air into just about anybody's day. Not all of us have access to such things though and may have to travel very far if we decided to get more in touch with the beauty of our natural world.

If you can't easily sperate yourself from the rat race and frantic trappings of an unnatural environment, if you can't easily go and get back in touch with Mother Nature, you can still bring her a little closer to you! Trust me when I tell you that she won't mind, and also trust that just by adding a few plants to your domicile can help to lower stress and even make your home healthier.

A less illustrated and chronicled reason for insomnia sneaking up on us may be related to the quality of our indoor air. If you can't properly breath during the night then getting to sleep will only be that much harder. Even if you are a devout neat freak an assortment of different molds and odors can start to grow within our homes and go unrecognized for far too long. These things can lower the quality of our air the same way that normal air pollution can. That's another one to watch out for, air pollution. It is probably seeping in from the outside and into your bedroom without you ever being the wiser to it. Yet research studies have shown, even a particular one performed by NASA, that plants can help to purify the air that we breath. Just simply being around plants, and taking the time to properly care for them, can induce a sense of wellbeing along with clearing out our airwaves. When it comes to reducing mental stress, one of the answers is literally all around us in the world of plants.

If you think that your trouble with sleeping at night is more mental than physical then you may want to start investing in some plant life and placing them all over your home. Specifically, place plants in the room that you normally sleep in. Going the extra mile would be to grow the plants from scratch inside your bedroom, but that may not be applicable for everyone, and understandably so. Even if it is not, don't fret. There are a large number of different plants that you can find and set down in your bedroom without having to grow them from scratch. Just remember to treat the plants with kindness and take care of them correctly, do not neglect them. After all, aside from being a part of Mother Nature, they are helping to calm your nerves and clear the air of toxins- both of which will help you sleep better at night.

Golden Pothos

This plant has also been called "Devil's Ivy" but don't let that trick you into avoiding it. This plant does have leaves that are slightly toxic, but it is also a very good plant to hang so it stays out of reach of children or animals. It is easy to care for however and is very handy at clearing out the air of pollutants. They can grow up to roughly around 30 feet indoors, so some pruning may be required. Within containers it shouldn't grow more than 10 feet. It has a vine, ivy, like appearance and is not susceptible to many pests, but every now and then may become infested with some bugs. It should be noted that the leaves should not ever be ingested.

Jasmine

This fan favorite has been shown to lower anxiety and promote better sleep. Using Jasmine plants to sleep better is nothing new and has been practiced for thousands of years. They also have glorious ivory or pink blossoms and are certainly easy on the eyes. They won't bloom at all if they don't receive enough cool temperature though, so keep that in mind. They also can, sometimes, grow rather wildly so pruning should be done regularly. Seeing as these plants can be enthusiastic climbers, an indoor trellis is recommended for them. They also are known to live for a long time when properly taken care of. They can be susceptible to infestation from mealybugs, keep an eye out for that.

Gerbera Daisies

It can be a bit difficult to not feel your spirits brighten when looking at this bright white, pink, yellow, and orange flower. They can also directly help to combat insomnia since during the night they release oxygen which will help to breathe easier. A word of warning is needed for these plants though; they are not the easiest to care for and not recommended to novices. They do require sunlight, but not direct or too much of it.

Seeing as how beautiful they are, it can be hard to not want to place them in your homes, but before selecting this plant do some extra research and make sure you can properly give it everything it needs.

Lavender

Many would consider this one to be the champion of the plant world when it comes to defeating insomnia. It has the double-edged power of both reducing anxiety and inducing sleep. It has been proven to slow the heart rate down and lower blood pressure as well. The scent of Lavender is world renowned, and for good reason. Simply smelling the delicate aroma may be all it takes to relax and ease into a better state for finding sleep.

Lavender is a moderate plant to care for. It may require pruning once a year and needs to be watered in different cycles relating to its age, but the benefits from making this plant one of your roommates can't be emphasized enough.

Snake Plant

Also known as "Mother-in-law's Tongue". That may be an odd nickname for a plant to have but don't be distracted by it. This is a great plant for beginners as it does not take much botanical knowledge to take proper care of it. They are also known to be hardy plants, so novices can be assured that even though they may be new to the world of living with plants, the Snake Plant will be able to endure whatever rookie mistakes they might make.

This should be one of your go to choices when choosing a plant to help alleviate insomnia. First, know that this plant emits oxygen during the evening hours which will start to clear the airways of where ever you slumber. Second, it also soaks up the carbon dioxide that is floating around us (carbon dioxide is something that we emit while breathing). Third, the Snake Plant has been proven to remove some of the common but unwanted toxins that are already floating through most homes such as; benzene, trichloroethylene, and formaldehyde. If all of that weren't enough, just know that a Snake Plant can be purchased already potted and ready to go. Sizes may slightly vary but acquiring a typical 6-inch potted Snake Plant should not be hard to find. All you have to do is find it, buy it, and set it. It is already to go right out of the gate.

Valerian

Pink, white, and the sweet scent of summer are just some of the ways to describe this plant. Even better, this plant has an ancient history when it comes to staving off insomnia. Galen, the famed Roman philosopher and physician, specifically used to prescribe Valerian root to rid his patients of insomnia. The modern research of today has caught up to Galen and promotes his claims from so long ago. According to some people, just inhaling the scent of Valerian root is enough to bring on a comfortable night of sound sleep. The herb of Valerian root will come in very handy when combating insomnia, but simply having a flower of it in your room can also kick your fight against insomnia into the next level. In the long-lost days were practicing magic was a common occurrence Valerian was used to construct dream pillows- just another cultural association between Valerian and getting some good sleep.

We could go all day about the different cultural and scientific links between Valerian and getting solid sleep, but it would take a whole entire other book to do so. It hasn't been labeled a medical wonder plant for no reason. All you should know before adding it to your living space is that it is a moderate plant to care for, so extra research may be required, and it is not recommended for people who spend a lot of time around horses, as it is not best for them.

Aloe Vera

This is another plant with a longstanding history in ancient cultures (it was dubbed by the

Egyptians as a plant of immortality). The plant has a cactus like appearance, but it is also one of the easiest plants to care for and is fine for novices. Although neglecting plants is not recommended, if your busy life causes you to forget to take care of your plant now and then, Aloe Vera will be able to handle itself just fine. It has a strong will to live and reproduces itself quite easily, so if you only start out with one then you will soon have enough to place in every room of the house, and maybe even be able to give away a few as surprise gifts.

NASA thinks very highly of Aloe Vera as well. They even went so far as to dub it one of the best plants to improve overall air quality. During the evening Aloe Vera releases oxygen into the air which will undoubtedly help you to get a better night's rest. If you are unsure which plant to get to help you sleep, don't want to take up too much space, or are lacking a green thumb, then this is certainly the one you should first add to your home and bedroom.

Precautions of living with plants

Although having plants in your home and bedroom can be very beneficial to reducing insomnia, there are a few precautions to keep in mind. If you have pets or children then make sure that the plants are not toxic to them. Knowing what is dangerous to certain animals, and your children's medical history, should always be first priority. It should also be mentioned that different people have different taste, so it is not just important to acquire plants whose appearance you appreciate, but also consider the aromas they give off and be sure that they are pleasurable to your sense of smell. You also will have to keep up with taking proper care of the plants, which involves a little bit more then watering them and making sure they get the proper sunlight. Be mindful to, at least once a week, clean the leaves by carefully wiping them. Making sure the leaves are clean will not just make the plants healthier but will also help them to do their job of keeping the air in your home purified. You help them, and they will help you, as goes the reciprocal balance of Mother Nature and all her precious children.

There are a number of different plants that can help to clean the air and bring on a better night's sleep but the once listed above are some of the best that you will be able to find without having to have a deep understanding of taking care of plants. Invite Mother Nature into your home and sleep easier after doing it.

Chapter 4:

The 10 Best Herbs for Sleeping Better

The world is overflowing with natural herbs. There are thousands, if not more, medicinal herbs in the natural world and these are the 10 best ones for getting better sleep.

Herbs, like modern medicine, do come with some warnings. If you are concerned with how these herbs may affect you, consult with your health care provider before taking any of these herbs.

These herbs are not appearing in any order of performance or superiority as not one of them is thoroughly better than any other. Use them one at a time or in conjunction with each other. Experiment and find out which ones you like best and help you the most.

Ashwagandha (Withania somnifera)

This herb is a part of the nightshade family. It originates from the dry regions of Yemen, China, and Nepal. It is a part of the species, *somnifera*, which can be translated to "sleep inducing" in Latin. The root powder of the plant has been used in traditional Indian medicine for centuries to combat several maladies, including insomnia. Modern scientific studies, including one done at the Sleep Institute in Japan, have confirmed that Ashwagandha does in fact bring about sleep, but exactly how and why remains unknown. Although exactly why Ashwagandha brings about peaceful sleep in unknown, it may have something to do with the water extract of the leaf being rich in triethylene glycol (TEG) which has been shown to reduce non-rapid eye movement (NREM). It has also been shown to reduce cortisol levels.

Ashwagandha should not be used by pregnant women. It may also aggravate symptoms of the following; thyroid disorders, lupus, multiple sclerosis, stomach ulcers, unbalanced blood pressure.

This herb is commonly consumed by brewing it in a tea. The standard dosage is 6000 milligrams a day (taken 3 times a day) or 100 milligrams when used in a cup of tea. It can also be purchased in supplement form.

Its appearance is orange or red, and a plum like bud.

California Poppy (Eschscholzia californica)

California Poppy is a resident of both Mexico and California. Also known as the "Cup of gold", this famed herb has even become the official state flower of California.

The side effects for using this herb to get over insomnia are minimal. It is still being researched how this herb may affect women during pregnancy, so it is better to avoid using it while pregnant. It also may slow down the nervous system too much, which is fine for sleeping but is not recommended for use if you have any sort of surgery coming up as it may conflict with anesthetics. Stop using this herb two weeks prior to any surgery. It should also be noted that the dosages for this herb can vary depending on age and other factors, so follow directions that come along with the herb carefully.

California Poppy has been shown to reduce a large collection of different nighttime aches while also slowing down the nervous system. These two factors combined can easily lead someone into falling asleep. Major ingredients within this herb are isoquinoline alkaloids. These alkaloids bind to serotonin and opioid receptors (this herb is not an opiate). Stimulating the opioid receptors is what blocks the pain and activating the serotonin receptors is what brings on the sleep.

It is commonly used in tea or can be purchased as an extract.

This herb has a very bright and sunny appearance, coming in different shades of yellow, orange, red, and on a rare occasion even pink.

Cordyceps (Cordyceps sinensis)

Cordyceps name is a combination of the Greek word for "club" and the Latin word for "head". Cordyceps are a fungus that grows all over Asia and have been used for medicinal purposes for ages.

Pregnant women should not eat Cordyceps. They can also, on rare occasions, cause diarrhea or upset the stomach but only when taken in large doses.

Cordyceps have been proven to dilatate the airways for our lungs, which allows more oxygen to reach our blood and induce sleep. Besides that, they also have shown to give boosts of energy and help athletes when training. Getting better sleep is only one of the benefits of eating Cordyceps. When taking them before bed they will induce a sedative like action and help to receive a deeper sleep. Seeing as this mushroom comes with a huge host of health benefits you should start adding it into your diet.

Cordyceps mushrooms are not known for tasting very good. When ingested they are usually powdered and dried out first. You can find them sold in jars and filled with powder, so they can be mixed with water, or you can buy them in the form of tablets.

German Chamomile (Matricaria chamomilla)

This one is well known and quite famous for helping people get better sleep. It has been used for centuries and found much popularity among the Greeks, Romans, and Egyptians. Its popularity hasn't dwindled either as this is still one of the most common herbs people reach for when trying to calm down and fall asleep.

A German study that tested Chamomile on animals showed that it acts as a mild sedative which helps to bring about sleep. A separate study researching Chamomiles affect against anxiety unveiled results that it reduces the symptoms of anxiety for people who have *generalized anxiety disorder* (GED). The gist is, lower doses of Chamomile reduce anxiety while higher doses induce sleep.

Do not ingest Chamomile if you are allergic to ragweed. Pregnant woman should avoid using Chamomile. It is also not recommended to be used in conjunction with NSAIDs (aspirin and other anti-inflammatory drugs).

Chamomile is typically used in a tea. There are a variety of different types of Chamomile that can be purchased and the two that you want to look for are Roman and German. We recommend using the German due to having our own better personal experiences, but that is subjective. Feel free to try both of them. It can also be purchased in capsule form, ointments, or the petals can be placed in bathwater.

Hops (Humulus lupulus)

These flowers are most famous for being used in beer and also being related to cannabis. It is not recommended to drink alcohol to reduce insomnia. You may fall sleep faster, but you may also wake up in the middle of the night. Although smoking cannabis may help bring about sleep, due to the illegality and controversy surrounding it, it is not recommended either.

Hops contain an active ingredient known as 2-methyl-3-buten-2-ol (MB). MB can interact with what is known as the GABA pathway. MB can bind with receptors in the brain and by doing so it can improve the binding of GABA. GABA is very important for falling and staying asleep.

People who suffer from insomnia have lower Gaba levels than those who don't. Hops also bind with our melatonin receptors. Melatonin is produced within our brains and is needed for falling asleep. It specifically produces itself when our eyes notice darkness and induces a sleepy feeling. By using Hops, you are binding to your GABA pathway and melatonin, getting a double whammy of neurological chemicals to help you fall asleep.

Pregnant women should avoid ingesting Hops. It should also not be used if you are currently suffering from depression. It may conflict with anesthetics. Stop using this herb two weeks prior to any surgery. It also contains some chemicals that mimic estrogen and as such should not be used for people who are dealing with hormone sensitive cancers or conditions.

An ancient practice using Hops for sleep was to make a pillow out of them. They are also brewed into tea, and in some cases even soft drinks.

Lavender (Lavandula officinalis)

Lavender is a native of the old world and grew almost on a global scale. Its gentle aroma is probably its most famous feature (next to its gorgeous violet appearance).

Several studies across the world have been done on Lavender in conjunction with sleep, although most of the studies were only small in scale. One study done in Thailand showed that Lavender may go so far as altering brain function to something calmer and more peaceful. It also showed a reduction in heart rate, respiratory rate, and blood pressure. Another research done in Britain specially relating to insomnia had several participants sleep in rooms where Lavender essential oil was pumped into the room while they slept at night while another group of people slept in rooms that did not have any Lavender. After a week of doing this the volunteers were polled on which rooms they received better sleep within, and 20 percent of them all agreed that the room with Lavender was superior.

Lavender is usually considered perfectly safe when ingested via the mouth. It should not be used by women who are pregnant or breastfeeding though. It is also not to be used by young boys who have yet to reach puberty, and it may conflict with anesthetics, so stop using this herb two weeks prior to any surgery.

There are a variety of different ways to use Lavender but it all comes down to the scent and oils. You can place a few drops of oil in a bath, place some of the flowers in a bowl next to your bed, put a few drops on your wrists or neck, spray it into the air before going to bed, or even sprinkle a tad of it on a tissue and place it underneath your pillow. Since Lavender is all about the scent, don't be scared to get a little bit creative with how you decide to use it.

Lemon Balm (Melissa officinalis)

Lemon Balm is a member of the mint family. It originates from parts of Asia, south-central Europe, the Mediterranean, and Iran. It has been used both to reduce pain and as a sleep aid ever since the Dark Ages

Lemon Balm contains something called eugenol. If you have ever been to a dentist then you have had this before, as it is what they use to numb a patient before doing work on the mouth. Eugenol is not just a numbing agent but can also help induce sleep. It is used to combat insomnia, and for people who don't have insomnia it is used to sleep longer. It has also been shown to reduce the symptoms of both anxiety and overall stress.

Lemon Balm should not be used by woman who are pregnant or breastfeeding. It also should not be used by people who have the following conditions; thyroid disease, diabetes, or anyone who has a surgery scheduled within two weeks.

Infants should not use Lemon Balm for more than four weeks. When taken by the mouth it may cause the following; dizziness, stomach pain, nausea, increased appetite. When applied to the skin it may act as an irritant.

Lemon Balm can be brewed in a tea (hot and iced are both used for Lemon Balm) but is also normally combined with Valerian root. While this herb can be used on its own, it is normally combined with other herbs and a variety of foods (it is a common and popular ice-cream topping). Candies, fruits, and even fish (have you ever eaten Lemon Balm pesto?) have been combined with Lemon Balm. A little extra tip when wanting to use Lemon Balm, mix it in a spearmint tea.
It can also be used for aromatherapy, as an oil, or applied externally.

Passionflower (Passiflora)

Passionflower can be found growing in Oceania, the United States, Southeast Asia, the Central and South Americas, and Mexico. This flower and vine is most known for producing the popular *Passion Fruit*. It also turns out that Passionflower has been used to treat several different health issues for many a number of years and between the 18th and 20th century it shot up in popularity and usage. Before that it was used by the Houma, Aztecs, and Cherokee people for fighting anxiety and getting better sleep.

It also has a rich, hidden, history. Legend says that while Spanish explores were adventuring through the Peruvian landscape they saw the Christian cross (Passion of the cross) hidden within the flower on multiple occasions.

Different studies have shown that by drinking Passionflower tea for 7 days may help to reduce anxiety as well as bring on a better night's sleep. This is another herb that can boost GABA levels in the brain, which is needed when trying to combat against insomnia. It has also been shown to relax nerves.

A study conducted in 2011 tested 41 participants by using Passionflower as compared to other items that can cause a placebo effect. Insomnia was one of the conditions that was specifically looked into. The results; those who used Passionflower claimed to have better results overcoming insomnia as compared to the other placebos.

In 2013 another study was done comparing three of the herbs in this list (Hops, Valerian, and Passionflower) against common pharmaceutical sleep aides. It was concluded that at the end of trial that the herbs did just as well, if not better, then the pharmaceutical drugs. Yet, none of the herbs showed to have addictive properties.

Stop using this herb two weeks prior to any surgery as it may conflict with anesthesia. Pregnant women should not use Passionflower. The effects of Passionflower while breastfeeding is inconclusive and thus should not be used. Also, when taken in large amounts, Passionflower may cause the following when taken via the mouth in large doses; nausea, inflamed blood vessels, an altered state of consciousness, confusion, dizziness, and irregular muscles action and coordination.

Passionflower is commonly brewed in teas. Most health food stores sell dried Passionflower and even already made, prepackaged, tea mixes. It can also be bought in capsules, tablets, and liquid extracts.

Siberian Ginseng (Eleutherococcus senticosus)

Everyone has heard of ginseng. The Chinese have been aggressively promoting the mountain sized list of benefits that ginseng offers to the human race for eons. The Russian people also have their own form of ginseng, and for ages it has been used to help people fall asleep. Just because it is also called "Devils shrub" should not scare you off from giving it an honest try. Also, be aware that

Siberian Ginseng is not a true ginseng, as it does not contain ginsenosides. Don't let that stop you either, as this herb has been labeled as a superfood.

Unfortunately, not many research studies have been done on Siberian Ginseng and its fame for reducing insomnia has spread more from word of mouth. That word of mouth has spread far though and in many circles this is one of the main herbs used to getting better sleep. It has also been extolled to fight off fatigue, boost energy, increase sexual functions, and is an anti-inflammatory.

Siberian Ginseng should not be used by women who are breastfeeding or pregnant. It also should not be used by anyone who has the following conditions; Diabetes, schizophrenia or mania, high blood pressure, heart conditions, cancer, or any bleeding disorder.

There are a huge number of different ways that you can take and use Siberian Ginseng. As with most herbs, it can be brewed in a tea on its own or combined with other herbs. You can also find it available as an extract, a supplement, a powder, or you can even find fresh Siberian Ginseng at a large variety of health food stores. If you have trouble locating it then check out some Asian food markets or order some online.

Valerian (Valeriana officinalis)

This lovely pink plant is a native to both Asia and Europe. Both the Romans and Greeks used Valerian often to combat against lack of sleep and lowering anxiety.

The National Institutes of Health have claimed that Valerian has a several different chemical compounds that work together to produce sedative properties. A separate group, the European Medicines Agency (EMA), approved of a health claim that Valerian can both produce sleep and act to reduce mild nervous tension when used as a dried extract.

Although exactly why Valerian works for battling insomnia is currently lacking clarity, it is most likely another herb that helps to increase GABA in the brain. It is believed that Valerian promotes GABA growth in two different ways. It may block an enzyme that destroys GABA, and by doing so more GABA can come in to help you fall asleep. The other thing that it is believed to do is release more GABA into your system. Not only is it producing more GABA, but it is blocking the forces that try to remove GABA. The hard science is still looking into this, but is it any wonder why Valerian has been used for besting the demon of insomnia for so long? In fact, even though many from the scientific community are still looking into the effects of Valerian, it is a common recommendation for weening people off of sleeping pills and falling back in tune with Mother Nature.

There is a window of time that should be taken into consideration when using Valerian though. 2-3 weeks are the magic numbers. Try using

Valerian for only 2-3 weeks, then take a break for another 2-3 weeks before starting to use it again.

Valerian should not be used by women who are breastfeeding or are pregnant. Its usage should also be stopped two weeks prior to any surgery. It is also not advisable to give to children who are 3 years old or younger. The rest of the side effects are minimal. It may cause any of the following; excitability, heart disturbances, mental dullness, dizziness, uneasiness, upset stomach, or headaches.

The part of the herb that is used to reduce insomnia is the root. Thankfully, there are several different ways to harness the power of Valerian without having to dig it up. As with most herbs it can be brewed in a tea. It can also be bought in the forms of capsules, tinctures, or tablets.

Chapter 5:

Herbal Teas

When dealing with natural herbs, the question of how to properly ingest them may arise. Different cultures that have relied on herbs for medicinal use, to overcome insomnia and other problems, have their own methods, opinions, and traditions. In some situations, the herbs have been either eaten or smoked. When dealing with insomnia and aiming to use herbs to fall asleep though, brewing them into a tea is a tried and true tradition that has not only withstood the test of time but is still being added onto in our current day and age. Modern research is constantly backing up what some of the ancient masters always knew and recommended; use tea to get better sleep.

Before turning in to go to sleep is the best time to

drink a cup of tea when using it to defeat insomnia. Different sources will give different directions for how to brew and drink it. It should go without saying, but the best way to brew your own tea is with a teapot, not some newfangled electronic device that will do all the work for you. It will be far easier for you to learn what works for you by doing it yourself. The thing to remember about tea is, it all comes down to the taste. You are free to alter these recipes and find out what works and tastes best to you.

There are two recommended ways to drink these teas after you brewed them. The first is to drink a full medium cup a half an hour before going to bed. The second is to drink several small amounts at your leisure several hours before bed. Experiment and see which method you enjoy more.

Unless otherwise stated, brew the teas listed here for 20 minutes after placing all the ingredients in. All water should be boiled beforehand. You can try to ice some of these teas if you want, but when doing so it will weaken the therapeutic effects and remember that a warmer body is more likely to fall asleep. Also, they really don't taste the same when iced.

All herbs should be strained before adding them to the tea.

There are a few light warnings to go over before diving into the different tea blends.

- Tea is not for young child. This is more or less a choice left up to the parents, but to be on the safe side, children should avoid partaking in stimulants.
- Tea should not be consumed by women who are currently pregnant.
- It is not safe to combine some teas and herbs with certain medications. If you are unsure, don't risk drinking any tea. Consult your doctor before doing anything else.

Easy Going Sleepy Time Tea Blend

This is sometimes known as "Simple Blend". It is an easy mixture that just about anyone will be able to brew even without having much experience making their own tea. As this is the first recipe there are not many details, you can add or take away what sort of herbs you want in it.

- 2 tablespoons of any sort of tea blend (non-caffeinated)
- 1 cup of boiling water
- Any amount and combination of strained herbs. The most common method is to use an equal amount of lavender and chamomile. Try one tablespoon of each and see how it works for you. If the taste doesn't agree with you, or if you don't receive the affects you want, try adding some different herbs, reduce the amount of either the lavender or chamomile, or increase one over the either.

Relaxing Tea Blend

This tea has a very interesting ingredient in it that I'm sure you will notice quickly.

- 1 cup of boiling water
- 1 teaspoon of catnip (yes people put this in tea, and have been doing so since the 1700's)
- 1 tablespoon of Valerian
- 1 tablespoon of Hops
- 1 tablespoon of Lemon Balm
- 2 tablespoons of Chamomile

Rest Easy Tea Blend

This tea is loaded with an assortment of different herbs to calm you down and rest easy.

- 1 cup of boiling water
- 1 and a half tablespoons of Hops
- 1 tablespoon of Passionflower
- 1 tablespoon of Oats
- 3 tablespoons of Chamomile

Miracle Tea Blend

This tea is a super sleep inducer. It will probably knock you out, but it has a heavy taste. Don't say you weren't warned.

- 1 cup of boiling water
- 1 tablespoon of Valerian
- 1 tablespoon of Lavender
- 2 tablespoons of Hops
- 3 tablespoons of Passionflower
- 3 tablespoons of Lemon Balm

Banana Cinnamon Tea

This tea is not a so-called herbal tea, but it is still all natural and will help calm you down to get the proper sleep you need. Ingesting some cinnamon can help even out blood sugar levels. Blood sugar, when too high or low, can disrupt part of your biological process and keep you awake longer then you want, or wake you up in the middle of the night. Another thing that you may not be aware of is that the peel part of the banana is actually loaded with magnesium and potassium.

The peel actually has more magnesium then the part of the banana that we usually eat. Both magnesium and potassium can help ease the muscles, which will help you get better sleep. This recipe also contains Stevia. Stevia will help to sweeten the drink and will also help balance out your blood sugar, and it won't spike your blood sugar before going to sleep. To top it all off, it is a unique tea, and is very easy to brew.

- 1 cup of boiling water
- 1 banana, with the peel. Cut both ends of the banana in half (the top and bottom) and toss them in with the water. Slice the peel up into several tiny pieces and toss them in as well.
- A pinch of cinnamon
- You should only boil this tea for ten minutes
- Add a pinch of Stevia
- Pour a cup and add more cinnamon if you desire

Chapter 6:

Naturally Beating Insomnia

When dealing with insomnia, taking in too much information at once can often seem staggering. For that reason, a comprehensive list of the top 10 best tips for beating your insomnia and getting back in tune with Mother Nature has been compiled for you. If ever confused, or just need a refresher, then simply just come back to this chapter and find out everything you need to know. Best of luck to you overcoming insomnia and reestablishing your relationship with Mother Nature.

Number 1: Use the herbs

Use the herbs in this book located in chapter 4. Learn more about them on your own and

experiment to see which ones work best for you.
Here are the best herbs used to beat insomnia;

- **Ashwagandha**
- **California Poppy**
- **Cordyceps**
- **German Chamomile**
- **Hops**
- **Lavender**
- **Lemon Balm**
- **Passionflower**
- **Siberian Ginseng**
- **Valerian**

Number 2: Drink Tea

Drink a cup of tea a day, preferably before going
to bed.

Number 3: Take Sleep Seriously

Understand why you have fallen into the pattern
of insomnia in the first place.

Number 4: Exercise and Meditate

Both of these activities will help to center both
the body and mind. They will also go a very long
way in getting your circadian clock back on its
proper track. Exercise will increase blood flow
and, when laying down to sleep, you will feel a
quicker sensation of sleep taking you over. By
exercising during the day, your body will better
understand exactly what muscles to restore and
functions to focus on while you sleep.

Meditation is the most natural method of clearing
up any mental issue, including insomnia. Not
only will practicing the different breathing
exercises help to control your heart rate and
increase oxygen, meditating (even for 5 minutes a
day) will also help to clear your thoughts and
organize all the action going on in your mind that
you were never even aware about. Although
exercise and meditation can give you a healthy
boost on their own, using them in conjunction
with each other is a formula that can't be beaten.

Just remember not to exercise too late at night, as that may keep you up longer.

Number 5: Melatonin and Magnesium

Most people don't realize that these two vital components that are needed for sleep are lacking in their bodies. Magnesium deficiency and a lack of melatonin being produced in the brain are more common than most people think. Check with your doctor to see if you are lacking either one of these, and then get a supplement to bring everything back in proper order.

Number 6: Sleep with Plants

Hang some plants in your home, especially the room that you go to sleep in. Doing so will not just clear the air, purify toxins, but will also replicate the great outdoors and you will be welcoming Mother Nature into your home with you. She is a fantastic roommate to bunk with.

Here is the list of plants to store in your home for quick reference;

- **Golden Pothos**
- **Jasmine**
- **Gerbera Daisies**
- **Lavender**
- **Snake Plant**
- **Valerian**
- **Aloe Vera**

Number 7: Read or Write in Bed

Writing and reading are the best activities to do before sleeping. Both of them will help to focus your mind while not placing it into a state of too much rapid thought. When doing either of these in bed, you are sending a direct message to your body that it is just about time to go to sleep.

Number 8: Get A Routine Before Bed

Creating a ritual and sticking to it, for about two weeks, will eventually cue your body that the time for sleep is approaching. You will notice that the longer you stick to the routine, you will start getting more tired before your routine has even finished. Taking a warm bath, then reading or writing in bed, are some great ways to get your nighttime routine started.

Number 9: Bright Days and Dark Nights

Emulate the sun and moon. During the day, surround yourself with light and try to remain active. During the night, lower the lights and slow down the energy. Also remember to kill off all electric lights (especially the blue ones) before going to bed. Keep in mind that your circadian clock will not reset itself all on its own. You have to be aligned with the sun and moon for it to return to its proper rhythm.

Number 10: Stop Reaching for The Pills

They may work in the short-term but when taken for too long they will only cause to increase your insomnia if you become addicted to them. Drop the pills. They are not one of the many gifts Mother Nature has bestowed upon us. Grab the plants and herbs, as that is what she has grown naturally on our planet Earth. To get back in touch with Mother Nature, use the resources she wants you to.

A final note

Now that you have gone through the entire book and reached the end you can stop and take a breather. Mother Nature will be very pleased that you have put in so much effort to learn more about her abundant bounty of heavenly and natural gifts. She has and will always be on your side. Yet, she is very busy trying to keep the planet (and the whole entire universe along with the spacetime continuum) alive at all times and, as much as you may not want to hear it, it is up to every single one of us as individuals to make the effort to stay on her good side. It is not up to her to come knocking on our door. No, it is the other way around. As it was already said, she will always be there for each and every single one of us, but we have to go to her.

Our modern day societies do not make this an easy task to complete. If anything, it seems like the runaround ways that society operates wants to keep us away from Mother Nature. This does not seem like it will change anytime soon either. So, as you partake in the herbs and get some well deserved better sleep, remember to keep up your effort to become closer to Mother Nature. By doing so, you will get a whole slew of other benefits then just better sleep out of it.

Conclusion

Thank for making it through to the end of *Herbal Medicine Insomnia: The 10 Best Solutions to Solve Insomnia Naturally*, let's hope it was informative and able to provide you with all of the tools you need to achieve your goals whatever they may be.

The next step is to get ready to do some shopping. Head on out to your local stores, or search online, and get your herbs ready to lead you into a world of sound sleep that you never knew of before! While you are out there grabbing your Lavender, Passionflower, Hops, and all the rest, be sure to pick up a few plants to hang in your home and bedroom along the way. Don't forget about making sure you have a teapot ready to go either or else when trying to brew some delicious and sleep-inducing tea, you'll be out of luck.

Start getting yourself, and your circadian clock, back in proper tune with Mother Nature and then you will wonder why you ever had problems sleeping in the first place. Just always remember that insomnia can sneak up on you again if you do not remain vigilant to keep it away. The herbs and tips in this book are not simply onetime quick fixes but long-lasting solutions that will continue to work as long as you continue to uphold them.

Rest easy and have sweet dreams.

Finally, if you found this book useful in any way, a review on Amazon is always appreciated!

This book belongs to a series of books about herbal medicine and how to use it to improve our life. For more information, visit www.db-publishing.com